THE HEALTHIEST SNACKS FOR ACTIVE KIDS!

Written By: Sam Hall

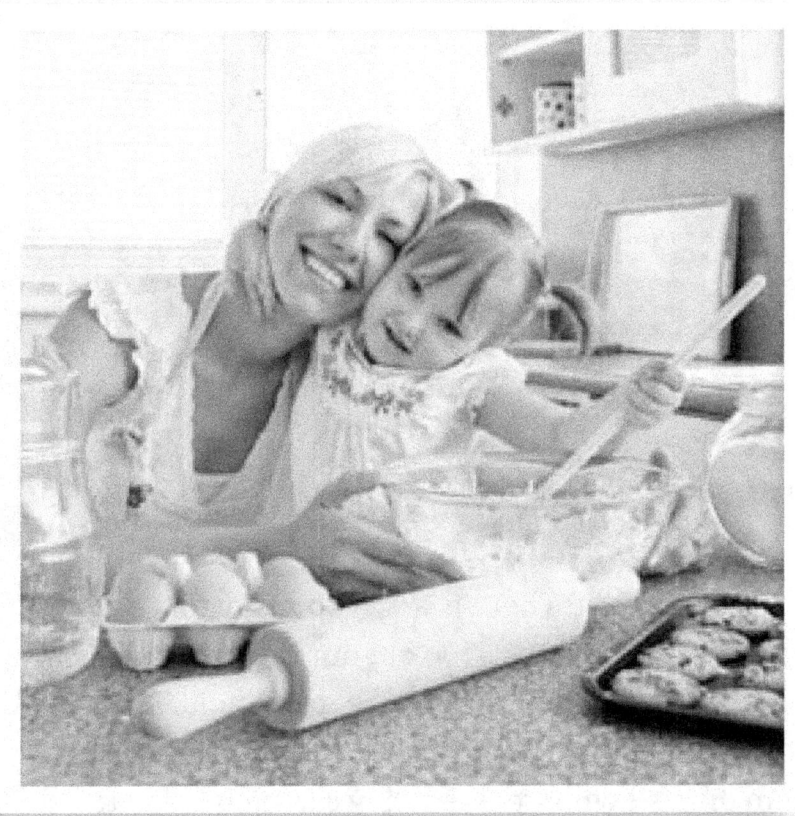

A mother's work is never done, and never is this more clear than when you finally exit the kitchen after post mealtime cleanup, only to bump into one of your little angels declaring they are so hungry! It's time to head back in and help them find a snack. With all of the other demands on your time, you're probably thinking that there are hardly enough hours in the day to keep them fed, much less tend to the rest of your commitments.

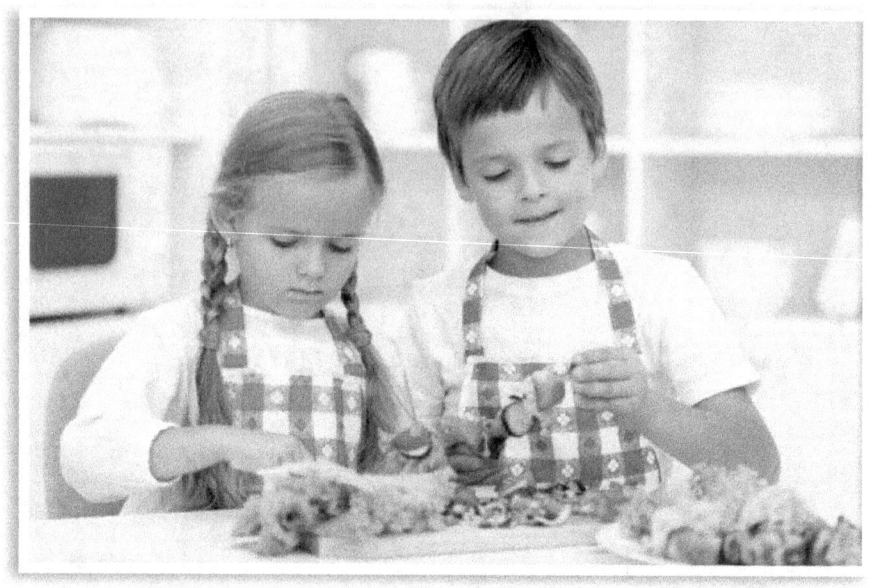

Take heart, lady! There is a way to make this easier on yourself. Simply take a look at our creative and healthy snack ideas and pick a few to keep on hand. If possible, store them in such a way that your kiddo might access them on his own, provided they can be trusted to ask permission. Then, you'll be able to simply answer they're I'm starving with Well, grab a snack!

GRANOLA BARS

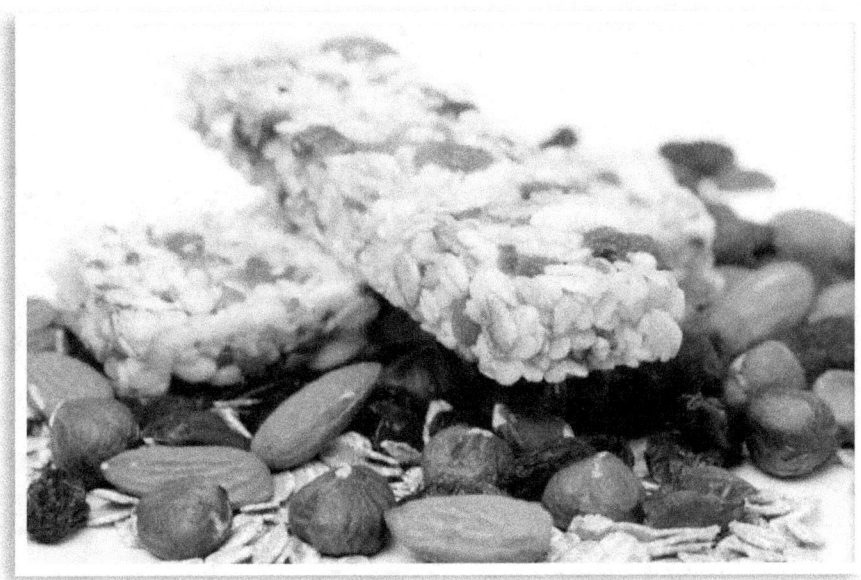

Multi-grain bars that incorporate dark chocolate, raisins, or bits of other dried fruits with some great nut protein are great to grab and go, so stock up on some good varieties on your pantry shelf. Make sure to pay attention to the added sugars, and try to select brands that specialize in whole grains and organic ingredients. If you're feeling especially Betty Crocker about things, you might try your hand at making your own homemade version.

CHICKEN SKEWERS

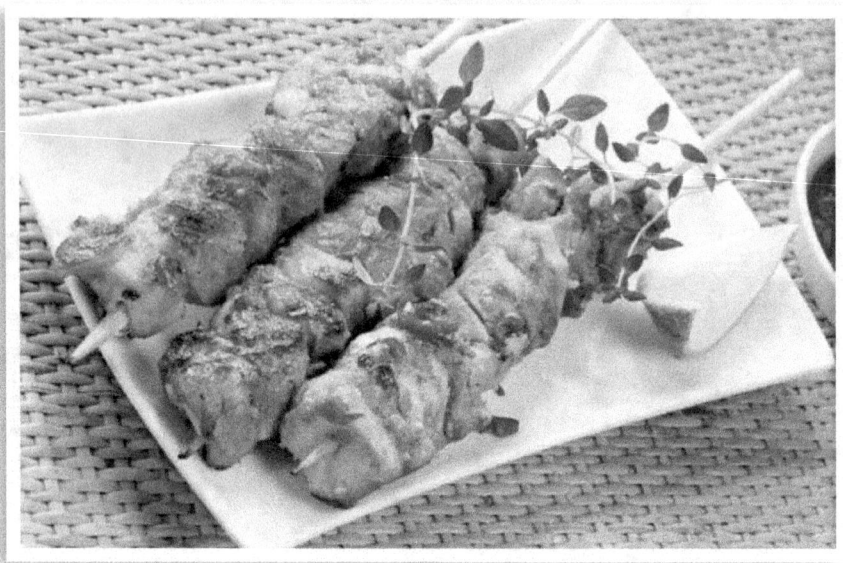

Kids love fried chicken fingers, but why not try getting rid of the breading and instead toss them on skewers with some honey or peanut sauce for flavor? They'll be getting a delicious chicken treat packed with protein, and you'll know that you kept them from consuming additional unnecessary fats. There's another bonus: much less oil mess to clean up.

SWEET POTATO FRIES

Slice your own sweet potatoes and bake them with minimal seasoning, and you've got a great alternative to traditional (and fattening) french fries.

FROZEN FRUIT

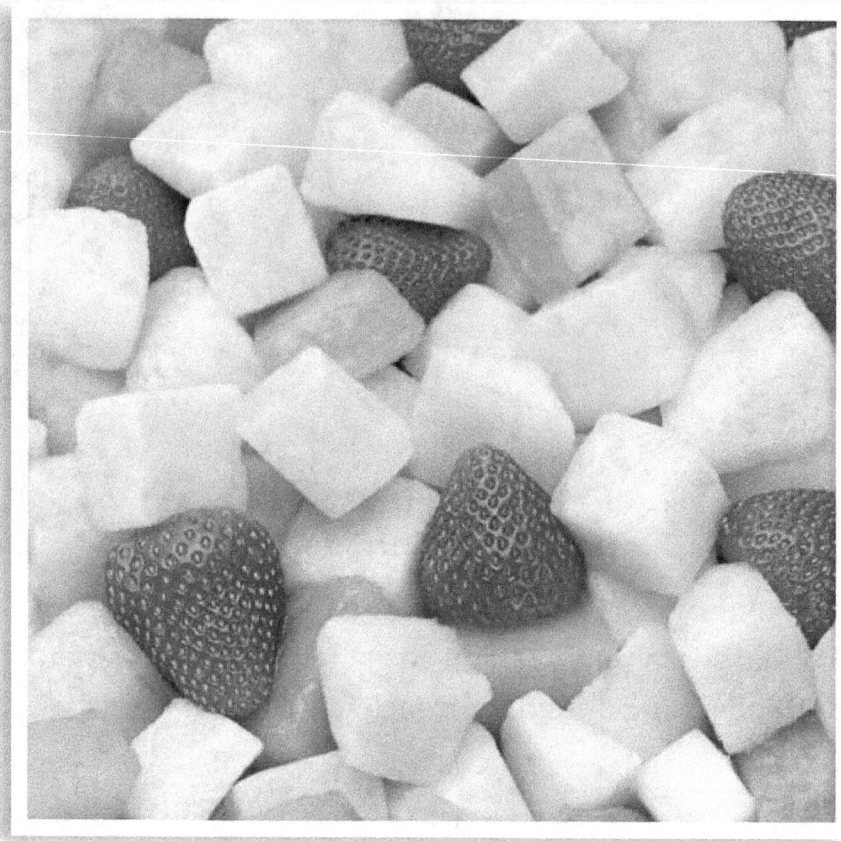

While we would all love to eat ice cream on these hot summer days, it's unfortunately not an option for daily consumption. Instead of ice cream, combine small bits of fruit into small containers and freeze. You can grab these on the way out the door, and in less than an hour you'll have a sweet and satisfying cool down treat.

CEREAL MIX

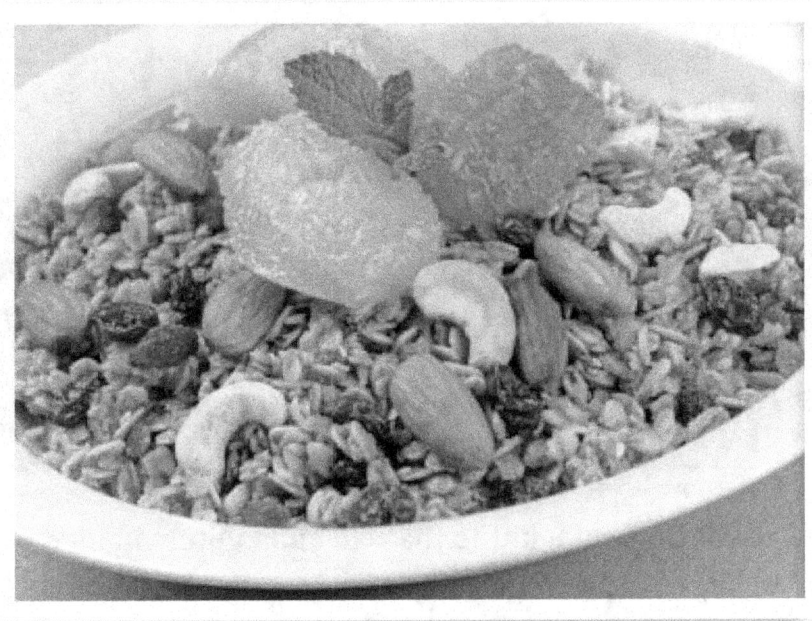

Grab a few different high fiber cereals to mix together in baggies that you can take with you. Add some nuts or dried fruit for a customized trail mix that the kiddos will love! This can get your kiddos hooked on walnuts or almonds, which are great for protein and healthy fats.

POPCORN

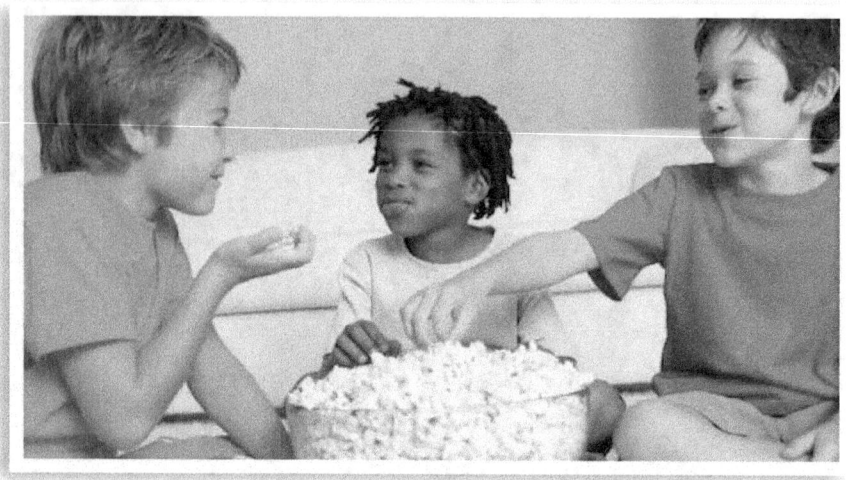

We've yet to meet a kiddo that isn't absolutely in love with the light yet satisfying crunch of popcorn. You can buy the microwave variety, just consider a low sodium low butter selection. Alternatively, you can pop your own kernels ahead of time and place some strategically in your bag and in the car.

NACHOS

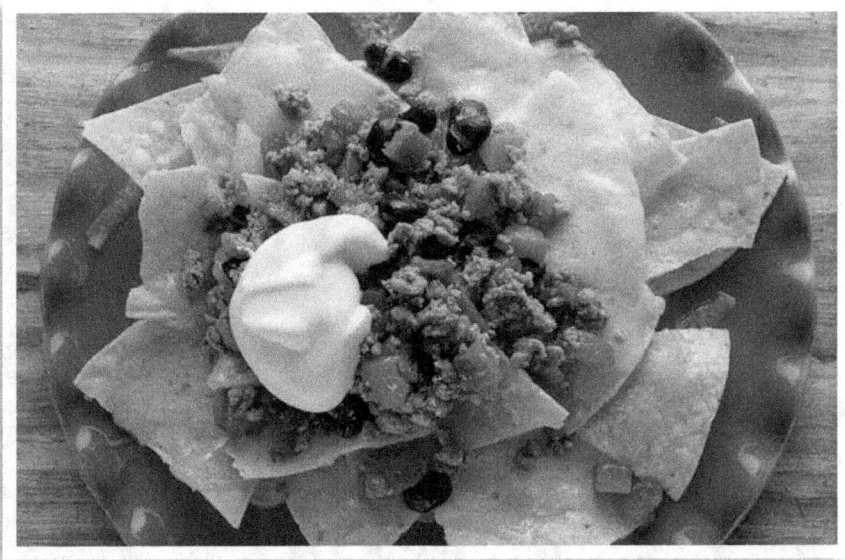

  Kid-friendly nachos couldn't be simpler to make. Turn on
the oven while your kids are piling up tortilla or corn chips
high with shredded cheese, then let them help you check
on their masterpiece as the cheese melts. You can try
serving with jalapenos or some salsa on the side if spicy is
on the menu.

FLAVORED MILKS

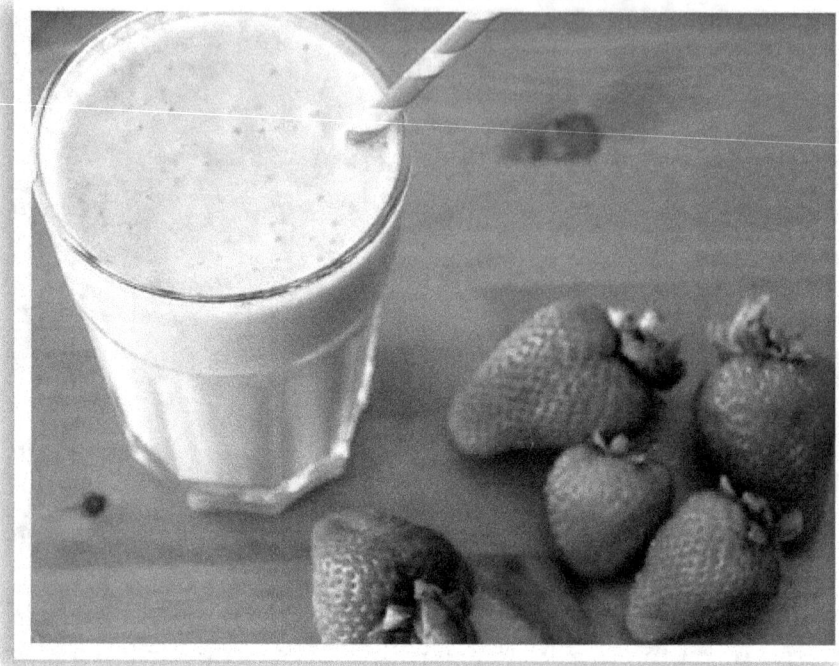

A dairy treat that doesn't involve ice cream and additional fat, you can still experiment with blending a variety of fruits directly into their low fat milk. This will make sure they get their daily supply of calcium, as well as some additional vitamins and minerals. These "milkshakes" are a great way to curb an appetite that won't wait for a meal that's not far away.

WHOLE GRAIN MUFFINS

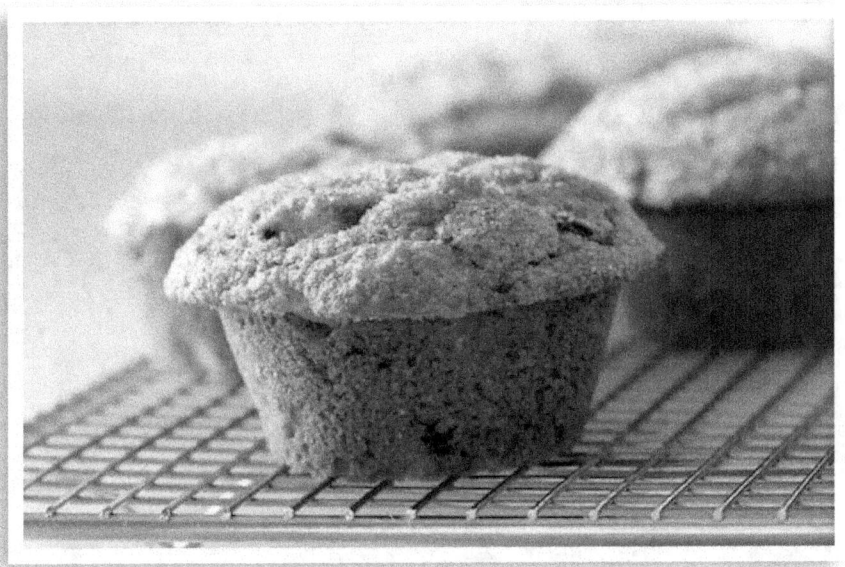

Make a few batches of whole grain muffins, with additional fruit and perhaps some nuts. These are great any time of day, not just for mornings. The individual portions will curb the tendency to over do it.

YOGURT PARFAIT

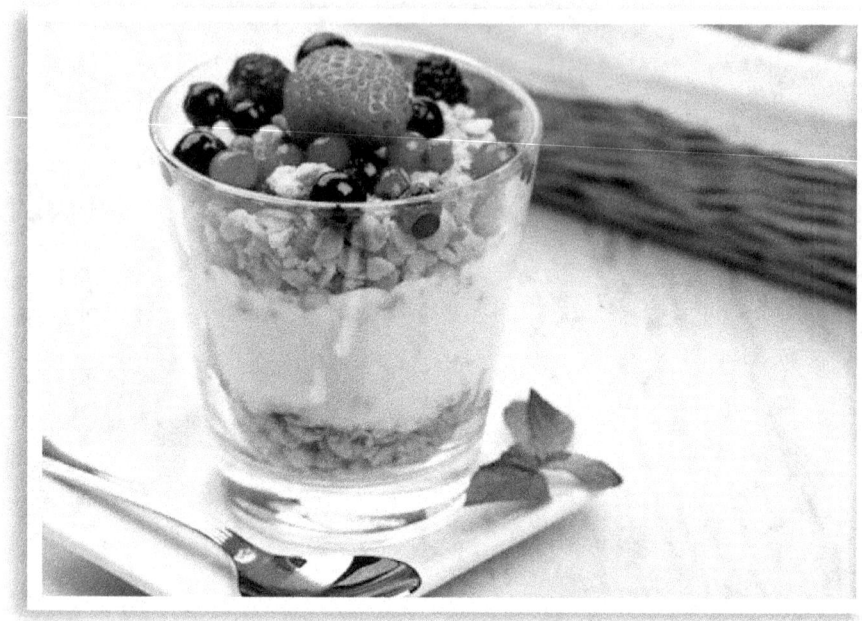

Layer fruit, granola, and yogurt to make a tasty and colorful treat that hits three main food groups at once, and is sweet enough to be a dessert. Keep a few of your kids' favorite fruits on hand for this, and start with lighter portions of granola. Eventually, they'll be gobbling up bowls full of this and asking for more.

PARMESAN CHEESE STICKS

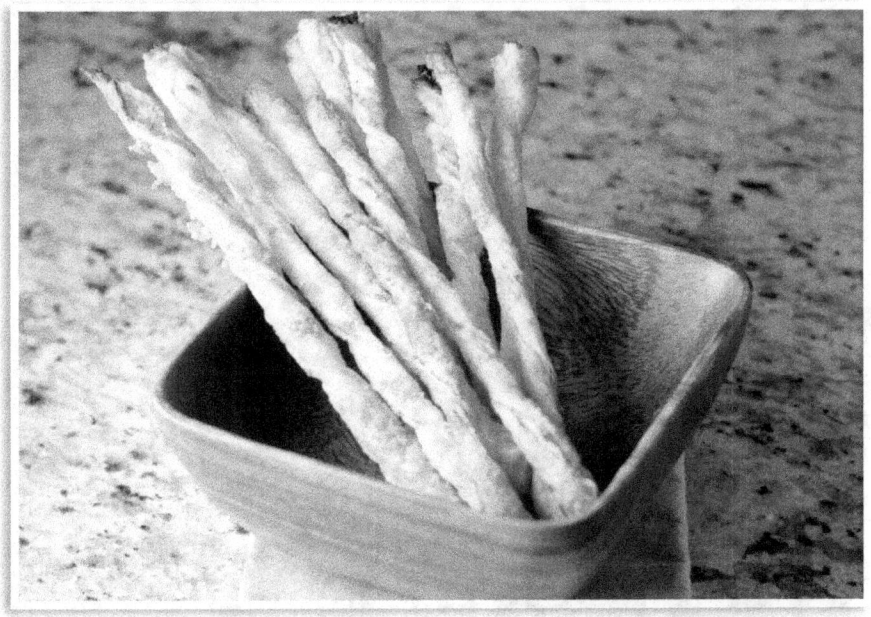

You can buy these or make your own, either way the cheesy goodness keeps the heavy carbs at bay. These are generally smaller than traditional breadsticks, so kiddos can enjoy a few of them without carbohydrate overload.

VEGGIE STRAWS

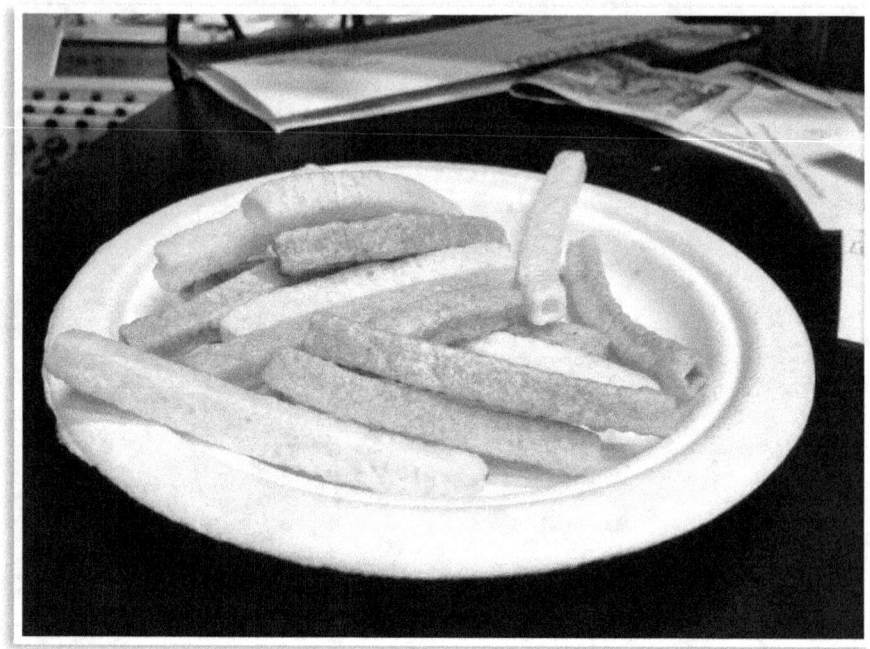

A satisfying crunch with delicate vegetable flavors, you can pick up a large bag of these anywhere. With a full serving of vegetables in every cup, you'll be happy to see your babes munching these down with abandon. Make sure to keep these individually portioned so you can snatch them on the way out the door.

JELLO SNACKS

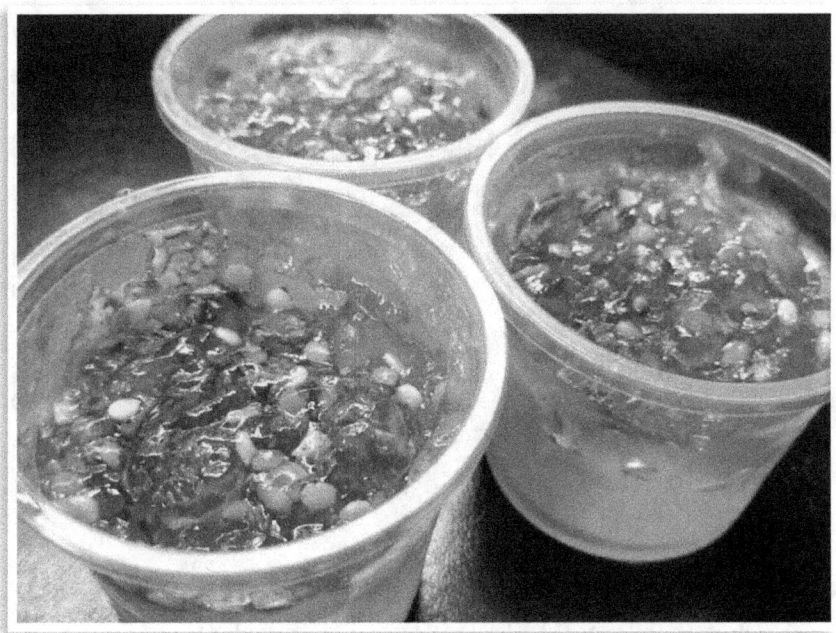

Mix a gelatin flavor with bits of fruit as it cools, and your kids will gobble up their fruit servings without a second look. Try different flavors, including peaches and pears. Best results can often be accomplished with canned fruit, so select some that is packed in water rather than syrup to minimize excess sugars.

VEGGIE STICKS

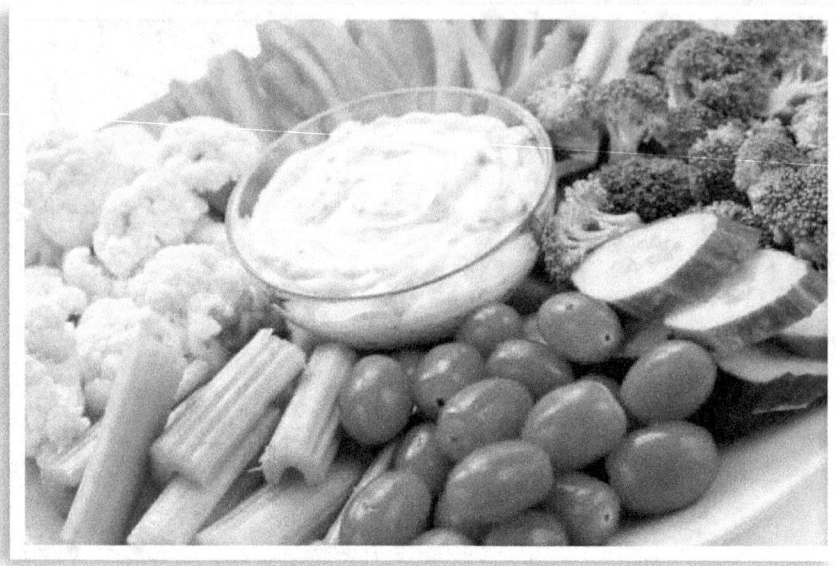

Any time you can trick a kid into eating his or her vegetables, you can declare a solid parenting win! The trick is to find a "dip" that your brood loves. Often, a little bit of peanut butter spread on an easy to manage stick form of carrots, peppers, or celery is the best route to take.

FRUIT DIP

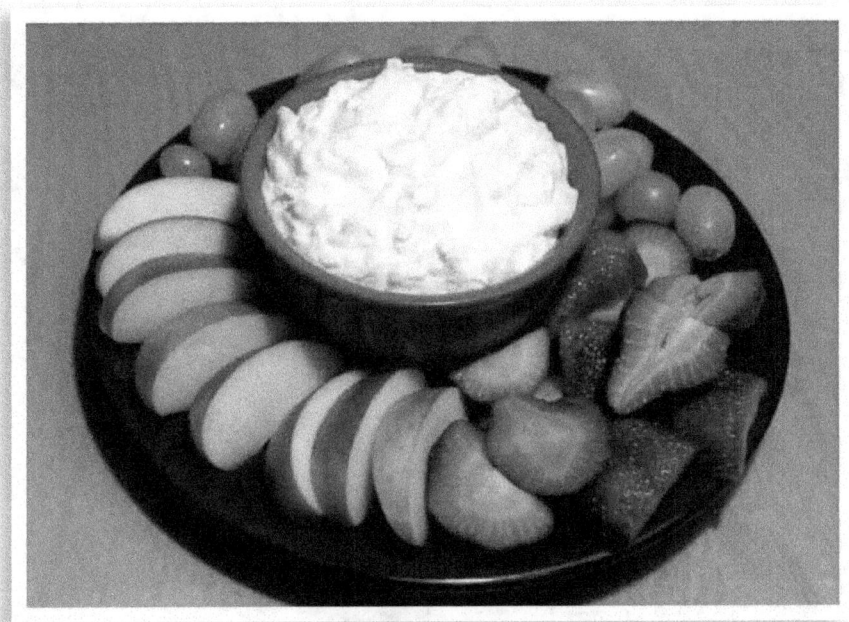

You can try the same trick with fruit, just make a cream dip that keeps well in the fridge and they can pull out on their own. You can also try caramel dip as an extra treat, but make sure that this happens only in moderation. You don't want to have kids bouncing off the walls from extra sugar when you just expected a sweet fruit treat.

CHEATER CHEESECAKE

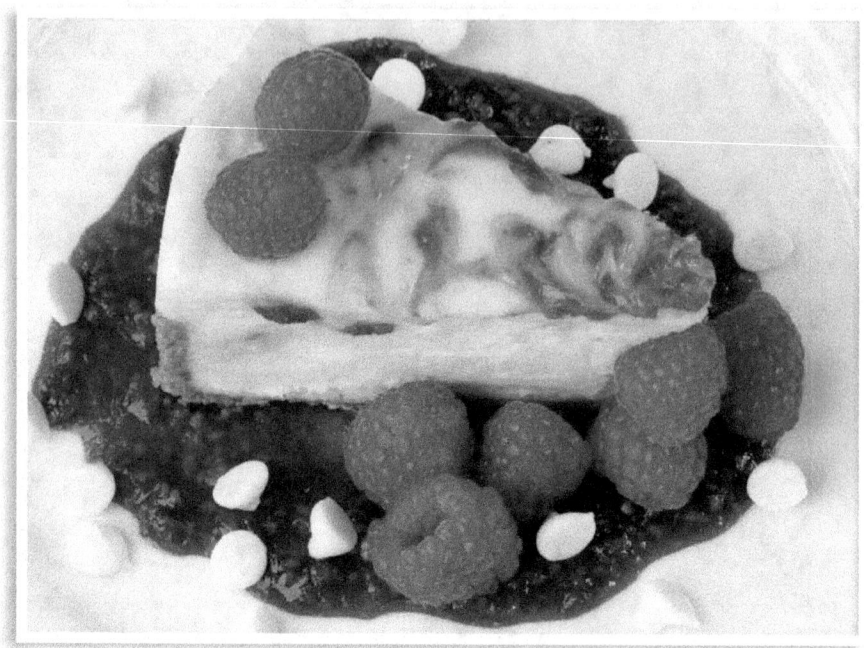

With a little softened cream cheese, some jam, and graham crackers, you've got a great approximation of cheesecake that the kids can help you make and enjoy in small portions. Mix in organic or local jam, and select multigrain grahams to maximize the nutrition. You can even top with sliced berries!

HOMEMADE POTATO CHIPS

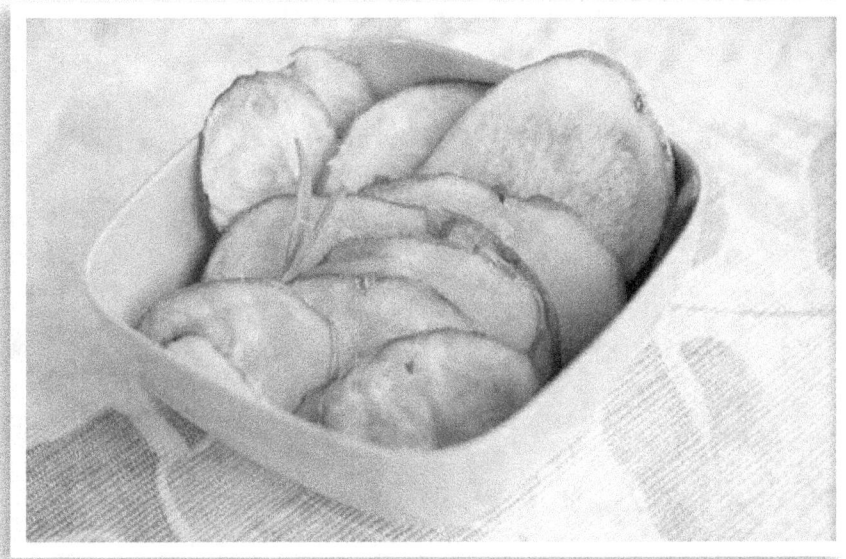

We cannot deny the lure of a delicious, deep fried potato chip. However, it's not the best alternative to always let the kids grab a bag full. You can teach them about where chips come from while serving a healthier alternative. Slice a potato thinly and spread over parchment paper with a small amount of salt. You can bake these in the oven, and voila! The perfect portion of homemade chips you can feel good about serving.

FRUIT CRACKERS

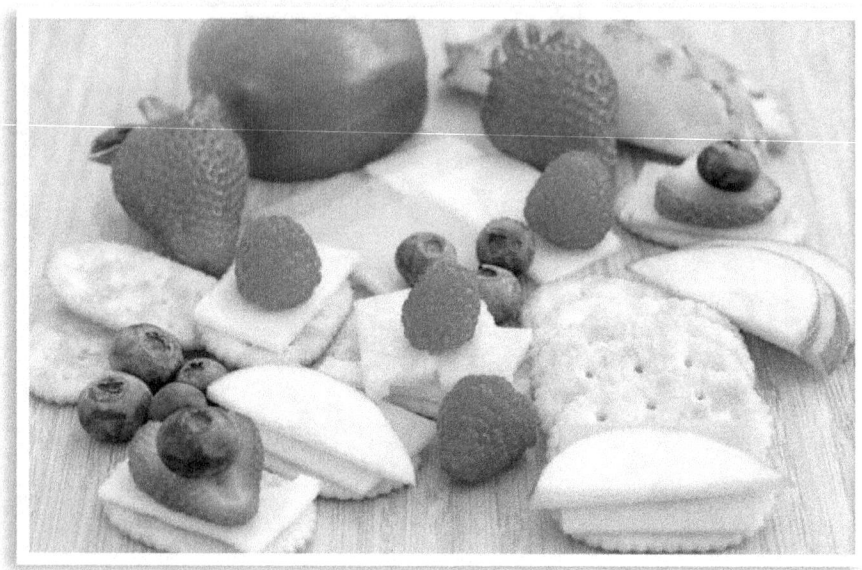

For a fall-flavored unique treat, choose a multigrain cracker to top with cranberry sauce and apple slices. Over that, add a touch of sliced cheese and broil until the cheese melts. It will taste like the fall air, and the fruit and cheese combination will make the kiddos forget about that whole grain goodness they are consuming.

Thank You!

We hope you enjoyed the book! All pictures and words were lovingly put together by experts who really love what they do! We really hope you learned something new today!

We would really appreciate it, if you could PLEASE take the time to let us know how we're doing by leaving a review on the Amazon website. We appreciate any comments you may have – what you enjoyed about the book, what additions you would have liked to have seen and what you would like to see in future publications.

Any comments will help understand better what you and your kids most enjoy and allows us to better provide exactly what you want!

Thought Junction Publishing

A NOTE FROM THE WRITER

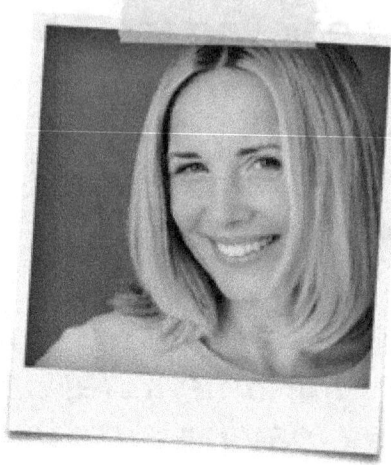

Sam's life revolves around her family, devoted mother of 3 - Noah (6), Oscar (3) and Poppy (11months) - she writes in a real way, aiming to answer the questions that other books don't cover, to fill in the blanks and inform parents and parents-to-be of the truth about raising children in the modern world.

Sam's writings emphasize that the readers are not alone - that there is a community of support available, and other people to talk to who can help, support and assist.

When she's not writing books, Sam is an advisor and avid blogger for Ideal Parent - http://ideal-parent.com - spreading support, care and advice across the web!

Join Sam on Ideal Parent and keep an eye out for her books - she's on a mission to help parents worldwide - join her and spread the word!